Contents

Acknowledgments

I would like to thank Joanna Pope, for all her invaluable help and advice.

My warmest thanks to David Simpson, for turning my typescript into an accessible guide and designing the supplement symbols used throughout the book.

Last but not least, special thanks to Alec, for all his practical help and support, and to all my family for their interest and encouragement.

Always consult your doctor if you are worried about any aspect of your health. The nutritional details in this book are for information only and are not intended to replace prescribed medications or medical advice.

Introduction

If you find the choice of health food supplements totally confusing, then this book is for you. It offers simple facts on vitamins, minerals, herbs and other nutrients, explaining what they are, how they work and the conditions they may help. It should enable you to decide what supplements to take to achieve your true health potential.

But, why do we need *any* extra nutrients? Surely a well-balanced diet provides all the ingredients necessary for good health without resorting to expensive supplements? In theory, the answer is probably yes, but in reality, our nutritional needs depend on our personal circumstances; what we eat and drink, our environment, health and lifestyle.

Let us consider the food aspect first. A 'healthy' diet is defined as one that includes plenty of complex carbohydrates (potatoes, wholemeal bread, pasta and cereals), lesser amounts of fish or meat, low intakes of fat and sugar and at least five daily portions of fruit and vegetables. Unfortunately, even with the best of intentions, most of us do not manage to eat nearly as well as this. Frequently rushed and short of time, we find ourselves relying on processed and 'convenience' foods which are quicker to prepare but may lack essential nutrients.

Many other factors deplete our vitamin and mineral levels, including pollution, modern farming methods, smoking, alcohol, stress and even drinking large amounts of tea, coffee and caffeinated drinks. Taking supplements remedies these nutritional deficiencies, whether their cause is environmental and beyond our control, or simply the result of poor eating habits.

We may decide to take supplements for a specific reason: to protect us against illness, to slow down the ageing process or to help overcome the effects of a particularly stressful time in our lives.

Supplements are natural nutrients, not drugs or instant cures. They are not intended to be a substitute for eating sensibly. Their good effects take time to build up, so it may be weeks or even months before we begin to feel their benefits.

So, in response to the question 'who needs to take supplements?' – the answer must be, that in today's busy and polluted world, we all probably do.

A word about RDAs

Recommended daily allowances for vitamins and minerals are set at the minimum level required to protect the general population against chronic deficiency. The term is misleading and RDAs should not be taken as a literal recommendation for individual nutritional needs. RDAs vary widely from country to country and do not reflect the level of nutrients required for optimum health. Research suggests we need intakes of vitamins and minerals significantly higher than RDA levels.

Simple explanatory terms
▼ Vitamins

Vitamins are organic nutrients that we need in minute amounts for healthy metabolism. They function closely with enzymes, controlling biochemical reactions within the cells and tissues of the body. With the exception of vitamin D, which the body manufactures after exposure to sunlight, we depend on our food intake to supply most of our vitamin requirements – and in theory, a well-balanced diet with plenty of fresh fruit and vegetables should provide all the nutrients we need for good health. Unfortunately, a significant proportion of the vitamin content of many foods is lost or depleted through storage, preparation, cooking and freezing.

Vitamins come in two forms – water soluble nutrients the body cannot store (B complex and vitamin C), and fat soluble ones (vitamins A, D, E and K) that remain in the body for longer periods.

Minerals

All our body minerals have come from food we have eaten. Minerals originate from the soil and are taken up by plants, which are eaten by us. Minerals may be lost in the preparation and processing of food – peeling vegetables and polishing rice, for example.

Like vitamins, minerals form two groups: the ones we need in large amounts like calcium and potassium are known as macrominerals; those we need in minute quantities are called trace elements.

Vitamins and minerals are measured in milligrams (mg) and micrograms (µg or mcg); a milligram is a thousandth of a gram, a microgram is a millionth of a gram. To add to the confusion, vitamin E is measured in international units (iu), 1mg = 1.5iu.

Herbal supplements

Over a quarter of all medicinal drugs in use today are originated or extracted from plants. Scientists are studying herbs that have generations of traditional uses behind them, and discovering important new powers in their active constituents. As well as treating health problems, herbs are becoming increasingly valued for their tonic effects. These work directly on the body's own healing system, boosting its ability to repair and regenerate itself.

Herbs are available in many different forms: as fresh, dried or packaged plants, or as convenient supplements, manufactured to pharmaceutical standards. Top brands like Solgar, apply stringent quality standards to their products, and are at the leading edge of scientific research into the amazing healing properties of plants and herbs.

Herbal supplements may be prepared from whole single herbs or combinations of herbs with complementary properties, or from standardised extracts. The latter are high-tech herbal supplements, offering exact amounts of specific plant compounds. Being uniform in quality they allow for the most precise dosing of the plant's active ingredients. Standardised extracts are more potent than whole herb products made from the entire plant, and many well-established herbs are now available in this format. Always check the label before buying.

Herbs are classified as supplements not drugs. Manufacturers are not allowed to state the conditions a herb can treat – which is confusing for consumers and one of the reasons for writing this book.

Other nutrients

In addition to vitamins, minerals and herbs, many other useful health supplements are available. These include fish oils, enzymes, hormones, amino acids, micro-algae, lactic bacteria products and various supplement combinations. These nutrients are described in the A to Z directory section.

Taking Supplements

Even when we combine a nutritious diet with a healthy lifestyle, we may still lack vital nutrients due to factors outside our control, like the stresses of modern living and a toxin-filled environment. Taking the appropriate vitamin and mineral supplements insures against any deficiencies and may help prevent serious disease.

Some people are more likely than others to be short on nutrients (especially trace minerals). Groups at risk include teenagers, pregnant women, the elderly, heavy drinkers and smokers and anyone on a restricted diet.

Health need	Suggested vitamin and mineral supplements
General good health	a quality multivitamin and multimineral (check label for ingredients)
Painful joints	cod liver oil, selenium
Premenstrual tension	B complex, vitamin B6, magnesium, evening primrose oil
Pregnancy and lactation	folic acid, calcium, quality multivitamin with maximum vitamin A content of 800µg
Menopause	B complex, vitamin C, vitamin E, calcium

Health need	Suggested vitamin and mineral supplements
More energy	B complex, vitamin C, co-enzyme Q10
Strong immune system	vitamins A, B complex, C and E, beta carotene, zinc, iron
Heart and circulation	B complex, vitamins A and E, beta carotene, calcium, zinc, magnesium, chromium, selenium, co-enzyme Q10
Stronger bones	calcium, magnesium, vitamin D, vitamin B6, boron, folic acid, zinc, copper, manganese
Vegetarian/ vegan diet	calcium, vitamin B12, iron, zinc, vitamin D
Cancer protection	vitamin C, vitamin E, selenium, zinc, copper, beta carotene, folic acid, vitamin B6, vitamin D, co-enzyme Q10
The elderly	vitamins A, B complex, C, D (taken as cod liver oil), E, calcium, selenium, co-enzyme Q10, iron

Remember...

■ Medications can deprive the body of certain nutrients: Antibiotics deplete vitamin B and the friendly bacteria living in the digestive tract; the contraceptive pill lowers levels of vitamin B6, vitamin C and folic acid. Over the counter indigestion remedies may interfere with iron calcium, vitamin A and folic acid absorption.

■ Drinking as little as three cups of coffee a day impairs the body's ability to absorb iron from food. Tannin in tea also inhibits iron absorption.

■ Caffeine in tea, coffee and soft drinks depletes potassium and other minerals through the urine.

■ If you don't exercise regularly you need extra calcium to keep your bones healthy.

■ Smoking (and inhaling cigarette smoke) more than doubles your vitamin C requirement (one cigarette destroys 25mg of vitamin C). Smoking also affects metabolism of vitamin B and is a contributory factor in osteoporosis.

■ Eat lots of vitamin-rich fruit and vegetables every day. Choose colourful vegetables and dark leafy greens to provide vitamin C, beta carotene, iron, calcium and folic acid. This is the best way to obtain and absorb these essential nutrients.

■ Wholegrains, wholewheat and unprocessed foods contain more nutrients than refined or processed foods.

Hints on choosing and using supplements

1 Buy well-known brands as these are manufactured to pharmaceutical standards and contain higher amounts of vitamins and minerals than cheaper supplements.

2 When buying herbal remedies, look out for products made from standardised extracts. These contain higher concentrations of the herb's active ingredients and are more potent than products based on powdered whole herb.

3 Always follow the directions on the pack and never exceed the maximum dose.

4 Store supplements in a cool, dry place and use by the best before date.

5 Most supplements are best taken with food to increase their absorption.

6 Vitamin E obtained from natural sources (labelled d-alpha tocopherol) is more effective than synthetic forms (labelled dl-alpha tocopherol).

7 Calcium supplements are better absorbed when taken with a milky drink at bedtime.

8 Most supplements must be taken regularly for one to three months before any benefits are felt.

The Really Useful Guide to Supplements

Vitamin A (Retinol)

A fat-soluble antioxidant nutrient that protects the body's cells against attack and builds up resistance to infection. Vitamin A is essential to the health of the skin and mucous passages and for good night-time vision. It may be prescribed as a cream or a high dose supplement to treat acne and psoriasis. Such treatments must always be medically supervised, as the body stores vitamin A and excessive intakes can be toxic. However, the . levels of vitamin A in fish oil supplements and multivitamin tablets are perfectly safe. Large doses of vitamin A should be avoided in pregnancy as they may cause foetal damage.

● Recommended daily allowance (RDA) 800µg (maximum intake from supplements should not exceed 2300µg).
Best food sources: Fish (herring, mackerel), meat (especially liver), eggs, margarine and dairy products such as butter and milk.

Acidophilus and Bifidus Bacteria

These are the names of two forms of friendly lacto-bacteria that aid digestion, protect the gut and help maintain the natural acidity of the vagina. Use of the contraceptive pill and antibiotics may deplete normal gut flora, causing an overgrowth of fungal organisms such as candida albicans and associated conditions like thrush. A course of acidophilus and bifidus bacteria helps restore a healthy gut environment. Supplements (usually tablets or capsules) should be kept in the fridge (to preserve viable bacteria) and are best taken after food with milk or yoghurt. Live yoghurt also contains useful amounts of lacto-bacteria.

Agnus Castus

A Mediterranean herb used to relieve symptoms of premenstrual tension and the menopause. The dried fruit's peppery aroma is thought to act on the pituitary gland and hypothalamus area of the brain, which control hormone production and activity.

Users of hormone replacement therapy and the contraceptive pill may find that the herb is not compatible with synthetic hormones, so should seek advice from a qualified herbalist or the manufacturers before use. Agnus castus is available as a tincture or in tablet form from health food stores and mail order suppliers.

Alfalfa

The sprouts of the perennial plant alfalfa, a member of the pea family, have become a popular health food in recent years. The leaves of the plant contain small amounts of minerals, proteins, vitamins and other ingredients which help to stimulate poor appetite and may reduce high cholesterol levels.

Dried alfalfa leaf is available as a tincture and in tablet and capsule form. The recommended dose is 500–1000mg dried leaf daily or 1–2 ml of tincture. Alfalfa extract should not be taken during pregnancy.

Aloe Vera

The transparent gel from the leaves of this succulent plant is a proven skin healer, and used extensively as an ingredient in skin creams and lotions. The gel's soothing properties are especially effective when used in aftersun preparations. Aloe vera can also be taken internally to improve digestion, absorption, and as a laxative. It makes a good tonic, as it has strong anti-viral properties to boost the immune system. A good selection of aloe vera products in liquid and capsule form is available from all health food stores and pharmacies.

Amino Acids

The body uses 21 different amino acids to build the proteins of the body that make up our tissues and organs. These are obtained from our diet when we digest proteins, or are made by the body. Amino acids help build the hormones that control the different body systems and also the enzymes triggering the millions of chemical reactions happening within us every second.

Research into amino acids is an exciting area of nutritional medicine, as each amino acid has its own therapeutic effects.

Eight are labelled 'essential', which means we must obtain them through our food intake because they are not produced in adequate quantities in the body, like the non-essential amino acids.

The eight essential amino acids are as follows:

■ **Isoleucine** – promotes skin growth

and healthy haemoglobin.

■ **Leucine** – promotes healing in skin and bones and lowers blood sugar levels.

■ **Lysine** – inhibits the growth of viruses and is needed by the skin for production of collagen.

■ **Methionine** – is involved in the manufacture of nucleic acid – the regenerative part of collagen.

■ **Phenylalanine** – regulates the thyroid gland and controls skin colouring. Used as an antidepressant, painkiller and appetite suppressor. Phenylaline supplements should be avoided by pregnant and nursing women.

■ **Threonine** – affects the neurotransmitters in the brain, helping to overcome depression. May also reduce allergy symptoms.

■ **Tryptophan** – used to make serotonin, a neurotransmitter that promotes sleep. Peanuts are a natural source of tryptophan.

■ **Valine** – regulates metabolism; acts as a stimulant so helps in alleviating depression; protects the myelin sheath surrounding the nerves in the brain and spinal cord.

Non-essential amino acids have an equally important role in maintaining health: **Arginine** and **Ornithine** stimulate muscle growth; **Carnitine** helps burn fat and build muscle; **Lysine** aids the absorption and utilisation of iron; **Glutathione, Cysteine** and **Taurine** are antioxidants; **Glutamine** builds up the immune system and is a tissue healer.

Amino acid supplements are available in 'free form' – that is, they are immediately used by the body and do not require digestion. They are a useful aid during periods of illness and convalescence, in old age, or during stressful or extra busy periods of life.

Caution: Amino acids should not be taken by children or during pregnancy. Seek advice before taking extra amino acids if you suffer from diabetes, hypertension, schizophrenia or take MAO drugs.

Best natural sources: Protein foods such as meat (especially pork and chicken), eggs, dairy produce, oats, eggs, beans, pulses, garlic, nuts and seeds.

Anthocyanidins

Anthocyanidins are nutrients found in small quantities in dark-skinned fruits. Their role in collagen production (the stretchy material in certain tissues) has been the subject of much scientific research. Collagen is responsible for the suppleness of the skin, and is found in high concentrations in the capillary walls.

Anthocyanidins taken on a regular basis maintain the health of these tiny blood vessels. They are similar in structure to bioflavonoids, but are more active and better absorbed and dispersed throughout the body. Anthocyanidins are powerful antioxidants, soaking up free radicals and helping the absorption of vitamin C.

Although these nutrients are found in many foods, cooking, freezing and preserving destroys them.

Anthocyanidin capsules are usually prepared from extracts of bilberry, grapeseed or pine bark and are available from health food stores and mail order suppliers. They should not be taken in pregnancy.

Antioxidants

These are important nutrients that protect body cells from the harmful effects of 'free radicals' (the highly unstable and reactive molecules created when oxygen combines with food to produce energy). Pollution, smoking, stress and other environmental factors all increase free radical numbers, causing damage to body cells and tissues.

The main antioxidant nutrients are vitamins A, C and E, beta carotene and selenium, all found in a healthy diet that includes fresh fruit and vegetables (five daily portions are recommended). Zinc, co-enzyme Q10, many herbal nutrients and amino acids also contain valuable antioxidant properties.

Busy, modern lifestyles, smoking, drinking alcohol, poor eating habits, illness and stress are all factors that may lead to a deficiency of antioxidant nutrients.

Taking a supplement safeguards levels of these vital nutrients, and should provide at least 150mg vitamin C, 100iu vitamin E, 10mg beta carotene and between 50–200 µg of selenium.

Best food sources: Fish, meat, eggs, dairy produce, bread, pasta and cereals, nuts, pulses, fresh fruit and vegetables.

Ashwagandha

One of the herbs used in traditional Indian (Ayurvedic) medicine as a tonic. Prepared from the roots of the *Withania somnifera* plant, ashwagandha is valued for its beneficial effect on the immune system, boosting the body's natural healing powers and improving skin and muscle tone. Like the herb ginseng, ashwagandha has a reputation for restoring male sexual potency.

The herb is relatively unknown in the West, but its reputation is growing. Capsules and extracts are becoming available in health food stores and from specialist herbal suppliers.

Astragalus

A herbal tonic prepared from the roots of the Chinese *Astragalus membranaceous* plant. Studies have confirmed that astragalus enhances the immune system by increasing the activity of white blood cells and the production of anti-bodies and interferon. It is a good tonic for people with chronic infectious diseases such as bronchitis and sinusitis, and for cancer patients undergoing treatment. Astragalus is also beneficial to anyone who is feeling debilitated by illness and lacking vitality.

Available from health food stores as a tincture or in capsules.

Vitamin B Complex

B complex vitamins are needed for the release of energy from food and the health of the nervous and digestive systems. They also help maintain healthy skin, hair and nails. These water-soluble vitamins cannot be stored by the body, so must be obtained from daily food intake. The complex consists of eight individual B vitamins: B1 (thiamin), B2 (riboflavin), B3 (niacin), B5 (pantothenic acid), B6 (pyridoxine), B9 (folic acid),

B12 (cobalamin) and biotin. Choline and inositol are related nutrients. B complex vitamins tend to occur together in food, although each has its own important properties and may be taken individually in supplement form. Heavy drinkers, the elderly, pregnant women, contraceptive pill users and those under stress have an increased need for B vitamins.

Supplements should include all eight B vitamins and provide more than 100 percent of the RDA for each one (the different levels and RDAs will be stated on the container). Since B complex vitamins tend to work together and occur as a group in the same kind of foods, taking individual B vitamins for specific needs may cause an imbalance. This can be avoided by taking a quality B complex supplement at the same time as the individual B vitamin.

Best food sources:
Wholegrains and cereals, milk, eggs, yeast, liver, meat, poultry and fish and leafy green vegetables.

■ Vitamin B1
(Thiamin)
Thiamin, the first of the B complex vitamins, is used by the body to release energy from food and to maintain the health of the digestive and nervous systems. As the body cannot store thiamin, it must be replaced by our daily food intake. Supplements (between 10–75mg) are most effective when taken as part of a good quality B complex preparation.

The elderly, smokers, alcoholics, contraceptive pill users, and anyone under stress or recovering from illness or surgery needs extra thiamin. The vitamin also helps prevent air and seasickness and some travellers find a 100mg dose is an effective insect deterrent.

● *RDA is 1.4mg.*
Best food sources:
Wheatgerm, oats, wholemeal bread, pork, hazelnuts, brewer's yeast and fortified breakfast cereals.

■ Vitamin B2
(Riboflavin)

Riboflavin is needed for energy release but is not easily absorbed by the body. A deficiency of riboflavin may cause irritating minor symptoms like itchy, dry, bloodshot eyes, cracked lips and mouth ulcers, which may be improved by taking 50–100mg daily. Riboflavin is used in food manufacture as a colouring. When taken as a supplement it is likely to turn urine a deep yellow; this is quite harmless.

● *RDA is 1.6mg.*
Best food sources:
Liver, cod and herring roe, mackerel, breakfast cereals, eggs and natural yoghurt.

■ Vitamin B3
(Niacin)

Niacin is the name for vitamin B3 and is found in two forms, nicotinic acid and nicotinamide.

Niacin helps maintain the health of the skin, mouth and digestive tract and is required for normal mental function and the release of energy from food. The body can make niacin from some protein foods. Best taken as part of a B complex supplement. Large doses of nicotinic acid, which must be taken under medical supervision only, can reduce high blood cholesterol levels but may cause facial flushing. If this is troublesome, Solgar make a 'no-flush' niacin supplement.

● *RDA is 18mg.*
Best food sources:
Liver, herring, mackerel, chicken, haddock, turkey and sardines.

■ Biotin
(also called coenzyme R or vitamin H)

Biotin is a separate supplement of vitamin B3, and essential for the normal metabolism of fat and protein. It has also been found useful in controlling overgrowth of the candida albicans organism. Biotin may prevent hair turning grey and delay balding in men, and is useful in alleviating eczema and dermatitis.

Alcohol, antibiotics, sulpha drugs, hormone replacement therapy and the contraceptive pill deplete biotin levels in the body; absorption is also prevented by the protein in raw egg white. So, if you drink alcohol or eggnogs regularly, or take the above types of medication, a 25µg biotin supplement is recommended. Biotin is found in most multi-vitamin and B complex supplements in doses of up to 300µg.

● *RDA is 150µg.*
Best food sources:
Offal, egg yolk, milk and dairy products, cereals, fish, fruit, nuts, cauliflower and mushrooms.

■ Pantothenic acid *(Vitamin B5)*

Another member of the B complex group and an important vitamin in its own right. Known as the 'anti-stress' vitamin, pantothenic acid has no known toxic side-effects and is widely available in many foods. It plays a vital role in releasing energy from food and helps to make anti-bodies to fight invading germs and bacteria. Pantothenic acid is also needed by the adrenal glands to help in the production of the stress hormone cortisone. Cortisone has a mildly anti-inflammatory effect, and supplements of pantothenic acid have been found to reduce pain and stiffness in some cases of rheumatoid arthritis. Supplements offer between 100–500mg daily. High potency 'slow release' forms are the best way to take this water-soluble vitamin.

● *RDA is 6mg.*
This should easily be obtained from the diet. Alcoholics and anyone under stress or using long term antibiotics may need considerably more than this.
Best food sources:
Liver, chicken, beef, yeast extract, eggs and dairy products.

■ Vitamin B6
(Pyridoxine)

Another important B complex vitamin often taken as a single supplement. Vitamin B6, is the 'anti-depression' vitamin, as it help to produce serotonin, a brain chemical which affects moods, sleep and behaviour.

Although vitamin B6 can be obtained from the diet, it is easily destroyed, as it leaches out into water during cooking and is sensitive to sunlight.

A daily intake of between 40–200mg vitamin B6 helps relieve premenstrual syndrome. The vitamin also protects against carpal tunnel syndrome (inflammation of the nerves passing through the wrist), reduces night muscle spasms and leg cramps and may prevent kidney stones occurring in susceptible people,

Hormone replacement therapy and the contraceptive pill may deplete vitamin B6 in the body, causing mild depression. This soon lifts when the deficiency is corrected. Safe and effective daily supplements provide between 50–200mg.

Following concerns that high levels of vitamin B6 caused nerve damage (peripheral neuropathy), over-the-counter sales of B6 in amounts over 10g in the UK were threatened. A campaign supported by leading nutritionists and scientists, convinced the Government that the research was incorrectly interpreted and that doses of up to 200–300mg daily are safe and should be available without prescription.

● *RDA is 2mg.*

Best food sources: Wheatgerm, oats, chicken, liver, fish, milk, nuts, soya beans, potatoes and bananas.

■ Folic Acid
(Vitamin B9)

Folic acid, as vitamin B9 is more commonly known, is essential for growth, cell division and the formation of haemoglobin in the red blood cells. It is vital for healthy foetal development and a minimum intake of 400µg is recommended for all women, prior to and during pregnancy. This will reduce the chances of having a baby with spina bifida, a condition in which the bony spine protecting the spinal cord fails to develop properly. Later in the pregnancy, folic acid helps prevent anaemia and extra is needed when breast-feeding.

Alcohol reduces folic acid's absorption from food. The contraceptive pill depletes levels of the vitamin in the blood; light and cooking also reduce folic acid supplies.

With the exception of pregnancy, folic acid is not usually taken as a supplement on its own, but is one of the nutrients in a multi-vitamin/mineral or B complex supplement.

Elderly people, smokers and drinkers usually have an increased need for folic acid. Supplements contain between 50µg and 400µg.

● *RDA in pre- and early pregnancy is 400µg, at other times 200µg.*

Best food sources:
Leafy green vegetables, brewer's yeast, nuts, wholemeal and soft grain white bread, liver.

■ Vitamin B12
(Cobalamin)

An essential nutrient for the normal metabolism of nerve tissue and for the healthy condition of the myelin sheath insulating the nerve fibres. Vitamin B12 is also necessary for the formation of healthy red blood cells and to give us energy. As the main source of this vitamin is animal products such as meat, liver, offal, eggs, cheese and milk, vegans and vegetarians may need a regular supplement to avoid becoming deficient. Algae, kelp and spirulina are good supplements for non-meat eaters as they all contain useful amounts of vitamin B12.

Like the other B vitamins, levels of B12 are depleted by heat, light, alcohol, smoking and the contraceptive pill. Alcohol drinkers and smokers need extra. The vitamin is non-toxic and can be taken safely in high amounts. An effective dose of vitamin B12 is 10–100µg taken at the same time as a good quality B complex supplement.

● *RDA is 10µg.*

Best food sources:
Meat, liver, offal, eggs, cheese, milk, yeast extract.

Bach Flower Remedies

The invention of Dr Edward Bach, an orthodox doctor and homoeopath who devised 38 plant and flower-based remedies to treat various mental and emotional states, each one being a complete system of healing. Safe, effective and completely natural, two drops of each required remedy is added to a glass of water and sipped. Bach Rescue Remedy is a unique combination of five flower remedies and is used by countless people in times of shock and emotional upheaval.

Bach Flower Remedies are sold in 10ml dropper bottles at health food stores and major pharmacies. Rescue Remedy is available in a larger size and in a cream form.

Beta Carotene
(see also Antioxidants, Carotenoids)

A unique nutrient that provides the pigmentation in plants (vegetables and fruits rich in beta carotene have orange, yellow and dark green colours).

Beta carotene has important antioxidant properties, which help 'mop' up excess free radicals in the body and protect the skin against ultraviolet damage. If our bodies need extra vitamin A, then beta carotene will be diverted into its manufacture, 1mg beta carotene making 167µg of vitamin A. Many vegans and vegetarians rely on beta carotene for their vitamin A intake. The nutrient is stored in fatty tissue in the body and is non-toxic in high intakes.

Beta carotene and the other carotenes found in

fruit and vegetables protect us against serious illnesses like cancer. For our health's sake, we should aim to consume at least five portions of fruit and vegetables daily, amounting to about 454g/1lb.

● *No RDA.*

A daily intake of around 10–15mg is recommended for optimum health.

Best food sources:
Carrots, tomatoes, spinach, broccoli, sweet peppers, watercress, cantaloupe melon, red and pink grapefruits, apricots, peaches, mangoes, and many other colourful fruits and vegetables.

Bilberry

A herb that offers useful natural help for eye problems and has been used successfully in clinical studies of various eye dysfunctions. It helps improve conditions such as macular degeneration, poor vision, glaucoma, cataracts and diabetic eye problems by strengthening the eye tissue and improving the circulation to the eyes. Its short-term effects on vision are most noticeable within the first four hours of taking it.

Bilberry extract is an especially rich source of anthocyanidins (special plant antioxidants) which have a positive effect on crucial enzymes affecting vision, and bioflavonoids (nutrients that increase the efficacy of vitamin C in the body). In addition to treating eyesight problems, the dried leaf is a traditional remedy for digestive disorders. Typical supplement range is 50–500mg daily (of standardised extract with 20–25 percent anthocyanidins). A non-toxic herb even when taken in large doses.

However, like most herbs with strong properties, it should not be taken in pregnancy.

Bioflavonoids

Also known as vitamin P, bioflavonoids are a group of phytonutrients (plant nutrients) found with vitamin C in fruit and vegetables.

Bioflavonoids increase the efficacy of vitamin C in the body, and act by strengthening the small blood vessels and speeding up healing of wounds, sprains and bruises. They help to maintain a healthy peripheral circulation, so are good for varicose veins. Rutin, hesperidin, citrin, flavones, flavonals and quercetin are all bioflavonoids.

Anyone whose diet is low in fresh fruit and vegetables, suffers from varicose veins or bruises easily, or who smokes or drinks alcohol will benefit from taking a supplement of vitamin C with bioflavonoids.

Blue Green Algae

One of the new 'superfood' supplements, loaded with antioxidants including amino acids, beta carotene, chlorophyll, vitamins and trace minerals. Recommended for anyone living a hectic modern lifestyle, as it provides valuable nutrition in an easily digested form. Klamath Lake blue green algae is a particular species of algae (*Alphanizomenon flos aquae*) found only in the mineral-rich lake in Oregon, USA.

During the 1996 harvesting season, another algae bloomed on Klamath Lake, producing toxins called microcystins, a known cause of liver damage. Some brands of supplements were later found to contain traces of this toxin. As a precaution, anyone buying Klamath Lake blue green algae should ask their supplier for an independent analysis of the product. The safety limit is one microgram of microcystin per gram of algae, assuming a daily supplement of two grams of blue green algae.

Borage
(Starflower Oil)

A rich source of gamma linolenic acid (GLA), an unusual fatty acid with no normal dietary source (the body makes it from linoleic acid found in vegetable oils).

GLA has a regulatory effect on the immune system, the circulation and the menstrual cycle. Interestingly, the chemical structure of borage (starflower oil) is quite different from that of evening primrose oil, another valuable source of GLA.

Borage (starflower oil) supplements may be taken singly or combined with evening primrose oil.

Boron

A trace mineral found in most plants and essential for healthy muscle and bone. New research suggests that boron supplementation may slow down calcium and magnesium loss from the bones of menopausal and post-menopausal women. Boron also benefits some forms of arthritis.

The mineral is included in many multivitamin and mineral supplements, or can be taken in the form of sodium borate to prevent osteoporosis.

Recommended dose is 3mg daily.
● *No RDA.*
Best food sources: Alfalfa, cabbage, soy, lettuce, peas, apples, dates, raisins, prunes, almonds and peanuts.

Brewer's Yeast

A cheap and natural source of B vitamins, but not as potent as a B complex supplement. Brewer's yeast is not recommended for thrush or candida albicans sufferers, or those with an allergy to yeast.

Bromelain

An enzyme found in pineapple that helps digest food and absorb nutrients. Available in tablet form from health food stores.

Vitamin C

Vitamin C – ascorbic acid – is a unique nutrient, essential to the health of the skin, hair, teeth, eyes, gums, bones and ligaments. Its main function is the repair and growth of body tissues and the maintenance of healthy blood vessels and red blood cells. The fluid between the cells contains vitamin C, enabling the nutrient to travel around the body fighting off free radicals and keeping the immune system in good order. Vitamin C is also needed for fat metabolism, to help with the body's absorption of iron, and to make collagen, a sticky substance that binds the cells together.

Unlike most animals which synthesise their own vitamin C, this water-soluble nutrient cannot be stored by the body, so we need a constant daily intake from our diet. Fruit, fruit juices and vegetables are all good sources. Vitamin C is highly unstable and easily destroyed by the processes of storing, peeling, freezing and cooking. To maximise the vitamin content of our food, we should buy fresh, seasonal produce whenever possible. Vegetables should be steamed or lightly cooked in small amounts of boiling water. As the vitamin dissolves in the cooking water, this should be used to make a nourishing gravy or soup.

Vitamin C is a popular and effective supplement to protect against colds and to speed up the healing process of wounds. Tablet and capsules are usually supplied in strengths up to 1000mg, and up to 5000mg per teaspoon in powder form. Look for supplements containing vitamin C with bioflavonoids, as these enhance the absorption and function of the vitamin in the body. If you need a less acidic, more gentle form of vitamin C, look for brands labelled Ester C™.

Although there are no proven toxic effects of vitamin C, excessive intakes are excreted but may occasionally cause diarrhoea, excess urination and even kidney stones in susceptible people.

● *RDA is 60mg.* Women taking the contraceptive pill, older people and smokers need considerably more than this – one cigarette destroys 25mg of the vitamin.

Best food sources: Fresh fruit, especially citrus fruits, kiwi, papayas, cantaloupe, blackcurrants, fresh fruit, strawberries, juices, green vegetables, tomatoes and new potatoes.

Calcium

The most abundant mineral in the body,

found in teeth, bones, soft tissues, nerves, muscles and blood. As well as creating healthy bones and teeth, calcium aids transmission of messages along the nerves and ensures muscle contraction. It helps the body to metabolise iron, promotes sleep, and keeps the heart beating regularly.

About 500mg of calcium is lost daily through the urine, so a regular intake of the mineral is needed every day from calcium-rich foods like dairy products, canned fish and dark green vegetables. Calcium deficiency causes leg cramps, and bone diseases such as osteoporosis and rickets.

When choosing a supplement of the mineral, look for preparations that include vitamin D, as this helps calcium absorption. For best results take calcium supplements with a milky drink before going to bed.

● *RDA is 800mg.* Teenagers, breastfeeding mums and older people need more.

Best food sources: Dairy products are the richest source of calcium in our diet, but the mineral is also found in eggs, canned sardines, tofu, nuts, spinach and bread.

Carotenoids

Carotenoids are coloured pigment compounds that occur naturally in fruit and vegetables – beta carotene being the most well-known member of the carotenoid family.

Although fruit and vegetables contain many different carotenoids, only about six are considered important for human health, protecting body cells and tissues from free radical attack. New research shows that some of the lesser known carotenoids such as alpha carotene, zeaxanthin, lycopene, lutein and cryptoxanthin may have even greater antioxidant properties than beta carotene, so a mixed natural carotenoid supplement is probably more beneficial than beta carotene on its own.

Beta carotene and certain other carotenoids also have the advantage of being precursors of vitamin A, that is they are converted into vitamin A by the body when needed.

To supply all the carotenoids and antioxidants needed to protect us against cancer and other illnesses, five portions (454 grams/1lb) of fresh fruit and vegetables should be eaten every day. Research suggests that the average diet is still deficient in these all-important foods. As our bodies find it easier to absorb nutrients from the diet, it makes sense to increase our intake of fresh vegetables and fruit rather than to rely on supplements to make up any deficiency.

Best food sources: Brightly coloured fresh vegetables and fruits.

Cat's Claw

A herb from the Peruvian rain-forest with unique properties that help increase the body's ability to fight and overcome harmful bacteria and viruses. Good as a tonic or whenever the immune system needs a boost. Available from health food stores and mail order suppliers as a herbal tea or in the form of a tablet or capsule containing a standardised full potency extract.

Chlorella
(see also Blue Green Algae and Spirulina)
A powdered food or tablet supplement, prepared from fresh-water micro algae and containing high levels of nutrients, including beta carotene, enzymes, vitamin B12, iron and selenium. One of the new 'green superfoods.' Available at most health food stores or through mail order suppliers.

Chlorophyll
The substance that makes plants green – found in the new 'green foods' such as algae, chlorella and spirulina. Chlorophyll is a rich source of magnesium and other trace minerals and has cleansing and alkalising properties.

Chondroitin Sulphate *(CSA)*
An amino acid related to glucosamine that is made naturally in the body and forms the main constituent of cartilage. Chondroitin sulphate allows other nutrients to pass through and nourish the cartilage structure, which does not have its own blood supply. Chondroitin sulphate and similar compounds are also present in the lining of blood vessels and the bladder, where they prevent abnormal components of blood or urine crossing vessel or bladder walls.

Recent research indicates that chondroitin sulphate may promote bone healing and help to restore joint function in osteoarthritis. Other studies suggest that it may favourably affect blood clotting, lower blood cholesterol levels and help prevent atherosclerosis (furring of the arteries).

Chondroitin's ability to be absorbed when taken orally is not fully understood and is still in doubt. Many nutritionists believe that when chondroitin sulphate and glucosamine sulphate are combined, they work synergistically to ease the pain of arthritis. New combinations of these nutrients have been promoted as a cure for arthritis in the US and are now available in health food stores in the UK.

Chromium

A trace mineral involved in metabolism and in particular with the production of insulin, the hormone made by the pancreas. Chromium lowers cholesterol and other fats in the blood, balances blood sugar levels and regulates the mechanism that controls appetite. The mineral has been shown to reduce body fat and increase lean muscle production in athletes. A deficiency may cause symptoms such as mental confusion, thirst, irritability, depression and problems with blood sugar levels leading to diabetes. Older people are more prone to chromium deficiency, as the ability to absorb the nutrient from food declines with age. Taking a chromium supplement may also help reduce sugar cravings when you want to lose weight, or have an addiction to chocolate, caffeine or cigarettes. Look for supplements labelled chromium picolinate, as this form is better absorbed and utilised by the body.

● *No official RDA level.*

Nutritionists recommend
25mcg. Supplements
offer 25–100mcg.
Best food sources:
Egg yolk, liver,
wholegrain cereals and
wheatgerm, yeast and
cheese.

Cobalamin
(see vitamin B12)

Coenzyme Q10
*(Also known as Vitamin
Q and Ubiquinone)*
A natural substance
found in all body cells
and used to 'spark off'
cell function and oxygen
utilisation. Coenzyme
Q10 also acts as an
important antioxidant,
stimulating white blood
cells to fight off
invading germs and
bacteria. Ageing and
environmental factors
decrease the body's
ability to produce
coenzyme Q10, causing
low energy levels
especially in older people.
Taking a supplement

may quickly improve
wellbeing and restore
energy levels.

Cardiologists have
also used coenzyme
Q10 with good results as
the nutrient helps to
boost the action of the
heart muscle. Another of
its benefits is that it
improves oral hygiene
and reduces gum
disease.

Most vegetarians, the
elderly, people who are
ill, low in energy, or
eating a poor diet are
probably deficient in
this important substance
and would benefit from
a daily dose of between
15–30mg.

Cod Liver Oil
(see Fish Oils)
Cod liver oil is the most
popular 'cold' weather
health food supplement
and a rich, natural
source of vitamins A and
D. It also contains some
essential fatty acids, but
in smaller amounts than

other types of fish oils. Cod liver oil helps maintain joint mobility and a healthy circulatory system and also helps to balance body calcium levels.

Available in liquid or capsule form; one-a-day capsules are especially convenient.

Copper

An essential trace mineral required in respiration to convert iron into haemoglobin. Copper utilises the amino acid tyrosine, allowing it to work as a pigment for the hair and skin. The mineral is also a vital component of many enzymes, including the antioxidant superoxide dismutase (SOD).

Copper deficiencies cause brittle bones but are unlikely in such a common mineral. Wearing a copper bangle allows traces of the mineral to be absorbed through the skin and is believed to ease joint pains.

Copper is found in most quality multi-vitamin and mineral preparations.

● *RDA is 1.2mg in Europe and 1.5 to 3mg in the USA.*

Best food sources: Nuts, wholegrain cereals, lentils, carrots, liver, crab and oysters.

Cranberry

The juice of this colourful red berry is a natural diuretic and urinary tract cleanser, helping to maintain health of the bladder, kidneys and prostate gland.

Research has shown that drinking cranberry juice lowers the pH of the urine and prevents the bacteria *Escherichia coli* (the cause of most urinary tract infections) from sticking to the bladder wall. Sufferers from cystitis or urinary tract infections (one in three women has this distressing problem at some time) may find drinking cranberry juice daily reduces the incidence of harmful bacteria in the bladder and prevents painful infections recurring.

Unsweetened cranberry juice (available in some health food stores) is the most potent form. Four fluid ounces daily is the recommended therapeutic dose. The unsweetened juice is too sharp for most people, who find the sweetened cranberry juice drinks and cocktails more palatable. As these are also more dilute, they must be taken in greater quantities to have a therapeutic effect.

You can now benefit from the cranberry without drinking the juice, as cranberry concentrate (in tablet or powder form) is now available from health food stores and pharmacies. It should always be taken with a glass of water.

Vitamin D

The 'sunshine vitamin' is so called because it is formed in the skin by the action of the sun on cholesterol. It is the only vitamin manufactured in the body, and plays an essential role in the function of the thyroid and parathyroid glands. Vitamin D also enables the body to utilise the minerals calcium and phosphorus, helping to build strong teeth and bones. Many calcium supplements include vitamin D because the vitamin aids calcium absorption. Rickets and other serious bone diseases are the result of vitamin D deficiency, but are now rarely seen, thanks to improved health care and the provision of vitamin D drops for babies.

As vitamin D is stored by the body, excessive intakes of more than 2000iu daily may be harmful. The maximum daily intake from supplements should not exceed 400iu. This allows for a more generous intake from the diet than most people achieve. Vegetarian vitamin D supplements can be obtained from health food stores.

● *RDA is 200iu.*
Breastfeeding women, the house-bound, vegetarians and those who have little or no exposure to the sun may need to take more than this.

Best food sources:
Oily fish (herrings, canned sardines and tuna), dairy products and margarine. Halibut liver oil and cod liver oil provide a rich natural source of this important vitamin.

Damiana

Damiana was originally grown for its medicinal uses in the hot climates of Central America. The leaves contain various active constituents (including essential oil of damiana) and have been used as an aphrodisiac since ancient times. Damiana is reputed to help sexual and hormonal problems and is also used as a sexuality tonic for women.

Supplements of the herb are available in tincture, tablet or capsule form. The usual dose is 400–800mg three times a day. Dried damiana leaves can be used to make a tea, also to be taken three times daily. Use one gram of leaves per cup and infuse for 10 minutes.

DHEA

Dehydroepiandrosterone (DHEA) is sold as an anti-ageing supplement in America and claims to slow down the biological clock and improve general health. It is also reputed to help weight loss (by speeding up the metabolism), to reduce pain and swelling in inflammatory joint disorders, and to protect against heart disease.

Natural DHEA is a male sex hormone produced in both sexes by the adrenal glands. Natural production of DHEA declines as we get older, leading to the familiar signs of ageing such as a spreading waistline, decreased energy levels and increased health problems.

Synthesised DHEA is available in America without a prescription and hailed as the new wonder supplement of the 1990s. Finding DHEA in Britain is more difficult, as the product is classified as a drug rather than a food supplement. Some UK health food stores will supply it on request and it is available by mail order on the Internet. DHEA can also be medically prescribed. Some doctors use it to treat menopausal women to reduce symptoms and improve libido.

Although the benefits of taking DHEA appear positive and exciting, the risks of taking such powerful hormones have not yet been fully researched and evaluated.

Devil's Claw

Devil's Claw (*Harpagophytum procumbens*) has been used by countless generations of native

Africans as a remedy for rheumatism and arthritis. The tubers are the only part of the plant that contain the active and curative phytosubstances in usable amounts. Devil's claw has been extensively researched, particularly in Germany. It has been successfully tested in various medical trials, confirming its effective anti-inflammatory properties.

For best results, an eight or nine week course of tablets is usually recommended to build up the active principles in the body, followed by a two or three week break.

The herb is available from health food stores and herbalists in the form of a tea, tablet or capsule. For best results only use products that specifically state they are prepared from only the secondary roots or tubers.

Although no side-effects have been reported from the use of this herb, diabetes sufferers are advised not to self-medicate with devil's claw.

Digestive Enzymes

Digestion and absorption are two of the most important physiological functions. If either of these processes are not working properly, our general health soon starts to suffer.

During the course of digestion, the body produces enzymes to break down food into molecules, small enough to be absorbed. Different types of enzymes work on different types of food – for example, protease acts on proteins, lipase on fats, amylase on starches. As we get older, production of these enzymes often declines, so that we are unable to absorb all the nutrients from food. Undigested or partially digested food passing into the lower gut is a common cause of wind and bloating. Many people, especially the elderly, find digestive enzyme capsules invaluable. They are available from health food stores and mail order suppliers.

DLPA

The abbreviated term for the combination of d-phenylalanine and l-phenylalanine, two amino acids involved in the body and mind's response to external influences.

Phenylalanine enhances the production of endorphins, the body's natural pain-killers. Endorphins elevate mood and reduce the sensation of pain. Phenylalanine is also a brain stimulant and involved in the manufacture of an appetite-controlling hormone called CCK (cholecystokinin).

DLPA supplements are quickly utilised by the body, so are useful for chronic pain control, to improve mental alertness and depression, and to control the appetite. Available as tablets or capsules from health food stores and mail order suppliers.

Dolomite

A magnesium carbonate supplement which helps maintain strong bones and a healthy heart. It reduces irritability and muscle 'twitching' and may be useful to women suffering from premenstrual syndrome and sugar cravings. Available from health food stores.

Dong Quai

Prepared from the root of *angelica sinenis*, a plant of the carrot family, dong quai has become a popular general tonic for women, helping relieve menstrual problems, hormonal imbalances, pre-menstrual syndrome and menopausal symptoms. In Chinese medicine, dong quai is also used as a men's tonic, as it is reputed to build muscle and blood. Although the herb is non-toxic, some women experience abdominal bloating or a change in their menstrual pattern when they first start taking it, but these symptoms soon pass.

Supplemental intake is usually 500–1500mg per day in capsule form; tinctures of dong quai are also available. Look for products that offer a guaranteed level of the herb's active ingredient, ligustilide. Dong quai is available from health food stores and mail order suppliers.

VitamIn E

This fat-soluble nutrient is stored and transported around the body dissolved in fats. Its powerful antioxidant properties protect the body against diseases associated with ageing, especially cancer and heart disease. Vitamin E helps maintain a healthy circulation by keeping the blood vessel walls clear and healthy, by preventing polyunsaturated fats from being oxidised into harmful saturated fats. Vitamin E is also needed for the synthesis of co-enzyme Q10, to improve the condition of dry skin, and plays an essential role in human fertility. Some women find taking a daily supplement of about 400iu relieves menopausal hot flushes. As vitamin E is stored in the body for only a short time (we lose more than 60 percent of our daily intake), we need a constant supply of this important antioxidant nutrient from food or through supplements.

Natural supplements (labelled d-alpha tocopherol) are generally more effective than synthetic ones (labelled dl-alpha tocopherol). In fact, natural source vitamin E is officially recognised to be over one-third more potent than its synthetic counterpart, and recent studies indicate that it is almost twice as effective.

● *RDA is 10iu.*
Much higher daily intakes (at least 50–80iu) are needed for the vitamin to have an antioxidant (protective) effect on the body.

Best food sources:
Vegetable oils, nuts, seeds and wheatgerm.

Echinacea

Processed extracts of this popular herbal supplement are derived from the roots and other parts of the purple coneflower, a member of the composite flower family, (which includes daisies, sunflowers and dandelions). Echinacea is one of the most widely researched herbs and has been found to be a rich source of numerous constituents that help support the immune system. Echinacea increases levels of interferon in the body and prompts the thymus gland, bone marrow and spleen to develop more of their immune cells.

The herb is most effective if taken for a couple of weeks when the immune system is under strain through illness, pollution or stress. Echinacea is available in tablet, capsule, drops or tincture form from health food stores and mail order suppliers. It should not be taken during pregnancy.

Evening Primrose Oil

The oil derived from the seeds of the evening primrose plant contains a special fatty acid called gamma linolenic acid (GLA). As there are no dietary sources of GLA, the body makes it from another fatty acid (linoleic acid), which is found in vegetable oils. GLA is used to make certain hormone regulatory substances (prostaglandins) which affect the immune system, circulation and menstrual cycles. Factors such as stress, alcohol, ageing, viruses and a lack of nutrients may block the body's manufacture of GLA. Evening primrose oil is a rich source of GLA and a safe and effective treatment for a wide range of disorders, including menstrual problems, rheumatoid arthritis, breast pain and certain skin conditions (it is available on prescription for atopic eczema). Its efficacy depends on the presence of certain other nutrients, so it is a good idea to link taking evening primrose oil with a multivitamin or to choose a supplement that also provides vitamin E. Therapeutic use of evening primrose oil is expensive, as quite large amounts have to be taken for several months before any benefits start to be felt. Effective treatment of conditions such as premenstrual syndrome require an intake of around 1500–2000mg, to be taken daily in the two weeks leading up to menstruation.

Evening primrose oil is a popular supplement and is available from health food stores, pharmacies, supermarkets and mail order suppliers.

Eyebright

As its name suggests, eyebright is a specific herbal remedy for eye problems. It is made into a tea or tincture, which is then used to bathe the eyes and eyelids. Eyebright has a drying effect, so is good for controlling hayfever symptoms. The herb is available as a dried extract, tincture, tablets or capsules from most health food stores and herbalists.

Fatty Acids

Although an excess of dietary fat is always undesirable, certain components of unsaturated fats are vital to health. These are known as 'fatty acids' and are found in fish and vegetable oils in two main groups Omega 3 and Omega 6 (named after their chemical structure).

Omega 3 fatty acids are 'sea' based nutrients found in fatty fish, fish liver oils and in limited amounts in some vegetables oils. The omega 3 group contains Eicosapentaenoic Acid (EPA) and Docosahexaenoic Acid (DHA). These two components produce prostaglandins, which reduce the stickiness of the blood, making it less liable to clot and cause thrombosis. By including oily fish once or twice a week in our diet, we can increase our intake of these important omega 3 fatty acids. They are known to lower blood pressure and promote a healthy cardiovascular system. Alternatively, a regular fish oil supplement has the same effect.

EPA prostaglandins are also thought to have anti-inflammatory properties that help to relieve an irritable bowel, psoriasis and arthritis.

Omega 6 fatty acids are 'land' based nutrients found in plentiful supply in vegetable oils. One of the key members of the omega 6 group is gamma linolenic acid (GLA), which the body generates from another fatty acid (linoleic acid) present in the diet. GLA is used to make prostaglandins, unique substances that regulate hormone production and the various body systems. Some people have difficulty converting linoleic acid into GLA, due to dietary or genetic factors. This may cause hormone-

related problems like premenstrual syndrome. Evening primrose oil and starflower oil are a direct source of GLA.

Best food sources
Omega 3 fatty acids: oily fish like herring, tuna mackerel and tuna. Omega 6 fatty acids: oils from cereals, pulses and vegetables.

Feverfew

This herb is a well-known natural remedy for migraine headaches. The leaves contain a substance called parthenolide which appears to inhibit the migraine-inducing negative effects of certain body chemicals like histamines and the brain chemical serotonin.

Feverfew is sold in health food stores in capsules, drops and tinctures. The average daily dose is 125mg. Quality feverfew products should be standardised for 0.1 – 0.2 percent of the active compound parthenolide. If the fresh leaves of the feverfew plant are eaten, they may cause a sore mouth and blisters on the lips.

Because of its effects on certain body chemicals, feverfew should not be taken by children, in pregnancy or by breastfeeding women.

Fish Oils
(see Fatty Acids)

A healthy diet should ideally include two servings of oily fish a week (salmon, mackerel, trout, herring, sardines, pilchards). Oily fish contains omega 3 fatty acids which help maintain a healthy heart and may ease painful rheumatic joints. For those who cannot eat this amount of fish, there are fish oil

supplements. These consist of two groups:
■ liver oils from white fish like cod and halibut;
■ fish oil concentrate from oily fish like salmon, mackerel, herring, sardines and pilchards.

Cod liver oil and halibut liver oil provide a rich source of vitamins A and D, helping to maintain healthy bones, skin, mucous passages and the immune system. Such oils contain only small amounts of omega 3 fatty acids, EPA and DHA.

Fish oil concentrate capsules contain negligible amounts of vitamins A and D but approximately 300mg of omega 3 fatty acids EPA and DHA per 1000mg capsule.

If an all-round supplement is required, combination fish oil capsules are available, or cod liver oil can be taken in liquid form as this contains high levels of vitamins A and D as well as omega 3 fatty acids.

Flax Seed Oil
(also known as Linseed Oil)

Flax seed oil is one of the richest sources of the omega 3 essential fatty acid alpha-linolenic acid. It also contains linoleic acid, an important relative of the omega 6 fatty acids, for which the evening primrose plant is cultivated. Research suggests that these important ingredients are essential for the maintenance of a healthy heart. Flax seed oil capsules are available from most health food stores. The recommended dose is 1 – 3 capsules daily. Whole or crushed flax seeds are high in fibre and add a nutty taste when sprinkled over cereals or vegetables. They have a laxative effect on some people.

Folic Acid
(see B complex vitamins)

Garlic

The cloves of this modest little plant have a strong odour and remarkable antiseptic properties. Over the years, garlic has proved to be an effective, natural protector against colds, catarrh and minor infections. Recent studies have shown that when garlic is incorporated into a healthy low fat diet, it thins the blood and reduces cholesterol and blood pressure levels. Garlic is also recommended for fungal conditions like thrush and candida albicans – cat and dog fleas also hate garlic! The herb contains various health-giving ingredients, the most well-known being allicin, a sulphur compound which forms when the cloves are crushed. This causes the enzyme alliinase to come into contact with alliin, a substance stored in the garlic cells. Allicin is what gives garlic its pungent smell, but disappears completely in cooking.

Fresh bulbs of garlic can be purchased from supermarkets and greengrocers. Garlic supplements come in various forms, including garlic oil capsules, tinctures and enteric coated tablets (which have a coating that prevents destruction of the active compounds by stomach acids). Supplements should always be swallowed with cold water at meal times, as hot drinks are likely to cause 'garlic breath'.

Genistein

An exciting new phytonutrient (plant) supplement derived from the soya bean. A distinctive feature of soya is its high isoflavone content (unique plant hormones that resemble the female sex hormone oestrogen but are only one-thousandth as potent). Isoflavones do not have an adverse effect as their oestrogen-like activity is very weak. They effectively block oestrogen receptors in the body by competing for sites normally occupied by oestrogen. This prevents hormone-dependent tumours flourishing.

In countries where the soya bean is a staple part of the diet, rates of breast, colon and prostate cancers are considerably lower. Soya isoflavones also may help to lower levels of cholesterol in the body.

Genistein is a well-studied soya isoflavone and anti-cancer agent. Extensive research suggests genistein prevents the growth of cancer cells in most forms of cancer; it inhibits the enzyme, tyrosine protein kinase, (known to stimulate cancer cell growth); Genistein may also help cancer cells return to normal; stop the growth of new blood vessels needed for a tumour to continue developing, and is a powerful antioxidant.

Genistein is now available in a tablet with another valuable isoflavone called daidzein, which is likely to improve bone density and prevent osteoporosis developing. This unique new supplement is available from selected health food stores or directly from Solgar Vitamins.

Ginger

Ginger is a spice obtained from the underground stem (rhizome) of the *Zingiber officinale* plant and is probably better known for its zesty flavour than for its health-enhancing properties. A popular ingredient in preserves, syrups and crystallised confectionery, ginger can also be eaten fresh, as the rhizome can be peeled, grated, chopped or squeezed for its juice. Ginger's therapeutic and warming properties have been valued since ancient times, especially as a remedy for digestive upsets, nausea and vomiting.

More recent research shows that ginger modifies certain chemical reactions in the body that cause abnormal inflammation and blood clotting. It tones up the circulatory system and helps to reduce the pain of inflammatory conditions like arthritis.

The spice also has important anti-cancer properties, preventing certain carcinogens from causing mutations within the body's cells.

Interestingly, ginger's complex chemistry undergoes changes when it is dried. Compounds called gingerols are converted into shogaols which have strong analgesic and anti-inflammatory effects. Capsules of dried ginger powder are therefore likely to be of greater therapeutic value to arthritis sufferers than fresh ginger.

The recommended dose is usually one capsule twice daily with meals.

Ginseng
(Panax Korean or American ginseng)

A herbal tonic prepared from the root of the ginseng plant and available in various forms, as capsules, tablets, powder, herbal tea, or even as a root for chewing. Korean and American ginseng belong to the *panax ginseng* species and should not be confused with Siberian ginseng, a completely different plant.

Panax ginseng contains a huge range of useful compounds that stimulate the nervous system and boost energy levels and alertness. These contain vitamins, minerals, hormones, amino acids and other nutrients. The herb maintains blood glucose levels and also helps to regulate blood pressure, so is useful in the control of diabetes. Ginseng's tonic effects boost the immune system and appear to have some anti-cancer properties. The herb is traditionally favoured by men and those who exercise regularly.

A note of caution: Because of the herb's natural hormone levels, ginseng should not be taken by pregnant women or women with breast disorders.

An average supplement dose is 100mg. To be effective, extracts should contain about seven percent of one or more ginsenosides (vital plant chemicals).

Ginkgo Biloba

Ginkgo biloba is prepared from leaf extracts of the *ginkgo biloba* tree, one of the world's oldest species. The Chinese have used ginkgo for thousands of years to treat many different conditions.

In the West, ginkgo has become a popular supplement because it may improve the circulation of oxygenated blood to the brain, legs, hands and feet.

The herb also has valuable antioxidant properties, improving mood and alertness in some people. A recent study of patients with Alzheimer-type senile dementia, showed that those who took ginkgo extract three times a day, showed a marked improvement in both memory and attention span.

Ginkgo is especially recommended for the older person. Not only does it aid concentration and memory, but the beneficial effects on the circulation ensure warmer hands and feet, relieving the cold fingers and toes experienced by many elderly people.

When buying a ginkgo biloba supplement, check that the product is standardised to contain at least 24 percent of plant chemicals called flavoglycosides.

Glucosamine Sulphate

An amino acid sugar formed from glucose and playing an important role in the making of soft tissue structures such as cartilage, tendons and ligaments. Age, injury and disease all deplete the body's levels of glucosamine, so injuries heal slowly, if at all. Glucosamine sulphate is a new supplement, developed to top up the body's production of glucosamine and speed healing of soft body structures. The new supplement has no adverse side-effects. It may help banish back pain, relieve arthritis and joint stress and promote the healing of sports injuries.

Golden Seal

A powerful medicinal herb prepared from the roots and rhizome of the *hydrastis canadensis* plant. Golden seal has a long history of use and a wide range of applications, being a particularly effective remedy for soothing digestive disturbances and nausea. It is also an efficient tonic for nerves, as it stimulates the central nervous system and endocrine glands. When made into a tincture or infusion, golden seal soothes eczema and other skin problems. It can also be used as an antiseptic mouthwash. The herb is an excellent remedy for all sorts of infections, especially those affecting the mucous membranes. It also helps to regulate menstruation.

Golden seal has a very powerful action and should not be used for prolonged periods or during pregnancy, as it may cause uterine contractions.

Gotu Kola

An Asian herbal remedy, valued as a natural treatment for varicose veins, lower leg circulatory disorders and to aid healing of skin and vascular tissue. Gotu Kola is also a useful diuretic, stimulates the central nervous system and may improve the memory. It has also been used to treat kidney stones, poor appetite, sleep disorders, fatigue and depression. Available from health food stores and herbal mail order suppliers.

Green Tea

The leaves and delicate young leaf buds of the bushy *Camellia sinensis* plant are used to make this health-giving drink. Widely cultivated in Asia, green tea contains numerous anti-cancer polyphenol compounds including the antioxidant flavonoid catechin.

Green tea numerous health benefits include-acting as a diuretic (used for years to alleviate the problem of swollen ankles); helping with weight loss by increasing metabolism of fat and regulating blood sugar and insulin levels; boosting cardiovascular health by lowering cholesterol levels; acting as a stimulant and reducing mental fatigue. Green tea's rich flavonoid content may also block the chemical reactions involved in producing allergy symptoms.

Recent studies indicate that green tea taken regularly may protect against cancers of the lung, pancreas, liver, skin and stomach.

This health-giving plant is available as a loose tea and in tea bags, with many grades and qualities to choose from. It tastes quite different from black tea, and for most people is an acquired taste. To enjoy the herb's therapeutic benefits, several cups of green tea must be consumed on a regular daily basis. Extracts of green tea are also available in capsule form. An average dose is 200mg (of an extract standardised for 25 percent polyphenols).

Green tea should not be taken by pregnant and nursing mothers. It contains caffeine (in smaller amounts than in black tea) so should be avoided by anyone with an irregular heartbeat or prone to anxiety attacks.

Green Lipped Mussel

Green lipped mussel extract is taken from a species found only in the unpolluted waters of New Zealand. When first introduced some years ago, green lipped mussel extract was hailed as the new arthritis 'cure'. Unfortunately, this proved to be an exaggerated claim, although some sufferers do find the extract helps their condition. Green lipped mussel extract remains a popular supplement and is taken by many people to maintain joint mobility.

Guarana

Also known as Brazilian cocoa, guarana is the legendary sacred fruit of the Amazon Indians and is popular throughout South America for the stimulant drink made from its roasted ground seeds.

Its anti-stress, tonic and diuretic properties are found helpful by people suffering from jet lag, nervous depression and hangovers. It is also used as an aid to concentration.

Guarana is available in capsule or tablet form from most health food stores.

Halibut Liver Oil
(see Fish Oils)

A well-established supplement which, taken regularly, protects the immune system and helps to keep teeth, bones and skin in good condition. Halibut liver oil capsules (and cod liver oil capsules) contain negligible amounts of omega 3 fatty acids EPA and DHA, but are a rich natural source of vitamins A and D.

Hydrochloric Acid *(HCl)*

Hydrochloric acid is produced in the stomach and is essential for the efficient digestion of food, especially proteins and vegetables. As we get older, we tend to produce less hydrochloric acid, although our need for it remains the same. Any deficiency means that food entering the intestines is not sufficiently acidic and too few enzymes are secreted by the pancreas for proper digestion.

Self-treatment with over-the-counter antacids for indigestion may worsen symptoms in the long run, as these further reduce the amount of acid in the stomach. Stomach acidity can be tested with specially coated capsules. Alternatively, seek your doctor's approval to take one or two betaine hydrochloride tablets with your meals daily to help digestion and improve vital nutrient absorption. Follow the directions on the pack and stop using the supplement if it causes any discomfort or burning sensation.

Hypericum
(see St John's Wort)

Iodine
(see Kelp)

A trace element essential for the formation of thyroxine and tri-iodothyroxine, the hormones manufactured by the thyroid gland which regulate the body's metabolism. An iodine deficiency leads to an underactive thyroid gland and many related problems, noticeably loss of energy, weight gain, dry skin, feeling cold and a slowing down of all body functions.

● *RDA is between 80 and 150µg (1µg per kilogram of body weight).*

Best food sources:
Fish, seafoods, garlic, watercress, seaweed, carageen and kelp.

Iron

A vital trace mineral used by the body to make haemoglobin, the red pigment of the blood. Haemoglobin is found in the red blood cells and transports the oxygen in the bloodstream around the body. Too little iron in the diet can lead to iron deficiency anaemia, which causes tiredness, lightheadedness and pale skin. Pregnant women (who have an increased need for iron), anaemic young women and vegetarians may need to take more iron than general supplements provide, so should seek a doctor's advice. Over-the-counter supplements are available in various forms. Choose organic iron compounds such as ferrous fumerate and ferrous gluconate, as these tend to be better tolerated than inorganic ones like ferrous sulphate, which destroy vitamin E in the body. Always check the label or ask advice before buying.

A unique and natural new way to take iron is in sachets of iron-rich spa water. Spatone™ is sourced from the iron-rich water of the Trefriw Wells Roman Spa in Wales and has none of the unpleasant side-effects associated with iron supplementation. It is sold in health food stores and pharmacies.
● *RDA is 14mg*.
Many people, especially women, need more.
Best food sources:
Liver, beef, eggs, dried apricots, wholemeal bread, fortified breakfast cereals, spinach, broccoli, potatoes and soya beans.

Vitamin K
A fat-soluble vitamin that plays an essential role in normal blood clotting, liver function and energising nerves and tissues. It is routinely given to newborn infants as a precaution against internal bleeding and may be prescribed for patients with liver disease. Vitamin K is not available on its own as a supplement, but may be included in some multivitamin preparations.
● *No official RDA*.
Best food sources:
Cauliflower and green vegetables, wholegrain cereals, kelp and alfalfa.

Kava-kava
One of the new herbal health supplements that have recently become available. Kava-kava

belongs to the pepper family (*Piper methysticum*) from the tropical islands of the South Pacific, where the root has been used for many years as an aid to relaxation and wellbeing. Kava-kava's relaxing properties are due to its oxygen-containing compounds known as lactones or pyrones, which have a safe and sedative action, and may act on certain neurotransmitters in the brain. Kava-kava is also a muscle relaxant and mood enhancer, relieving feelings of anxiety and depression.

The herb's popularity is growing, and supplements of kava-kava extract are available as tablets, capsules and tinctures. An average dose is 200–250mg of an extract standardised for 25–35 percent kavalactones.

For more refreshing sleep, cut out sugar and caffeine and take a kava-kava supplement combined with 500mg of magnesium.

Kelp
(see Iodine)

Kelp is the name given to various seaweed species, found on the coasts of Europe and North America. Kelp is a rich natural source of sea minerals, particularly iodine, the important trace element found in thyroxine, the hormone manufactured by the thyroid gland. Kelp tablets are popular with slimmers, as they stimulate a sluggish thyroid gland and speed up metabolism and the burning of calories. Three kelp tablets daily provide between 140–400 µg of iodine. Kelp should be avoided by pregnant women and those being treated with thyroxine. Always check with your GP if you suspect that your thyroid is underactive.

Lactic Bacteria

(see Acidophilus)

These 'friendly' micro-organisms transform sugars into lactic acid by a process called fermentation. In the human gut, these organisms assist food digestion and maintain a healthy acidic micro-environment. This protects the gut from harmful bacteria and the overgrowth of fungal organisms like *candida albicans*. Lactic bacteria is widely used in the food industry for the production of dairy goods such as 'live' yoghurt and other fermented milk products.

Lecithin

Lecithin is made in the liver and is found in all body cells, with large concentrations in the brain. Its role is to maintain the structure of the cell membrane and to aid the transportation and digestion of fat within the body.

Lecithin is a rich source of choline and inositol, nutrients related to the B complex vitamins that play an important role in fat metabolism. Choline is transformed into the brain chemical acetylcholine and is needed for normal brain activity and the transmission of messages between brain cells.

High lecithin intakes may slow down brain changes in the elderly and remove excess fat accumulation from the liver. Taking extra lecithin may even reduce the risk of gallstones in susceptible people, as it improves the bile's capacity to emulsify cholesterol. Lecithin also helps to preserve the myelin sheath which insulates the nerves and becomes depleted in multiple sclerosis.

Lecithin supplements (usually prepared from soya) are sold as tablets, capsules or granules. The granules may be sprinkled on food and provide higher intakes for specific health problems, one tablespoon being equivalent to about seven capsules. Even high intakes of lecithin are perfectly safe and have had no reported side-effects.

Magnesium

This mineral is a vital component of bones and teeth, helping the body utilise vitamins, calcium and other minerals. When it is combined with vitamin B6, magnesium ensures that calcium is deposited in the bones and not in the kidneys or blood vessels. The mineral is vital to many enzyme reactions in the body and is closely involved in energy release and the correct functioning of the nerves and muscles. As a natural tranquilliser, magnesium is useful in the treatment of epilepsy and premenstrual syndrome.

Deficiencies may cause irritability, anxiety, facial twitches and muscle spasms.

Magnesium is one of the most difficult minerals for our bodies to absorb from the diet. Supplements supply between 50–200mg per tablet or capsule, and may be combined with vitamin B6, or with calcium and vitamin D (when taken for bone health). Supplements sold for the treatment of premenstrual syndrome often include magnesium.

● *RDA is 300mg*.

Best food sources: Brown rice, wholemeal bread, brazil nuts, potatoes, peas, apricots and raisins.

Manganese

A trace element essential to the function of the pituitary gland (which controls normal growth and development), and also for brain, nerve and muscle action throughout the body.

Manganese is vital to the body's antioxidant defence system, as it is a component of an enzyme called superoxide dismutase (SOD), which fights free radicals and helps the body utilise vitamins B and C. The body needs manganese to make interferon, a natural anti-viral agent. The mineral is also involved in reproduction and the manufacture of breast milk.

Manganese is usually taken as part of a multivitamin and mineral preparation, in strengths of 5–100mg.

● *No RDA.*

Best food sources:
Almonds, wheatgerm, oats, wholegrain cereals, beetroot, beans, plums and pineapples.

Melatonin

Melatonin is a naturally-occurring hormone secreted in the tiny pineal gland in the brain. It responds to light through the eye and regulates the body's internal clock. As we age, the pineal produces less and less melatonin.

In the USA, where melatonin is sold as a nutritional supplement, the hormone has been hailed as a miracle 'cure-all', to banish insomnia and jet lag, boost immunity, prevent cancer and, most lucratively, to reverse the ageing process. Although some of these health claims may be exaggerated, the hormone appears to have many positive health benefits.

Melatonin is classified as a medicine rather than a food supplement in the UK, and is not available over the counter. If you want to try it as a remedy for sleeping problems or jet lag, buy it in the USA or ask your doctor for a prescription.

Milk Thistle

This thorny, spiny plant *(Silybum marianum)* has long been used to treat liver ailments. The seeds contain silymarin, an antioxidant plant chemical with powerful liver-protective properties. Silymarin enhances the metabolism of liver cells, protecting them from the effects of alcohol, heavy metals, drugs and other toxins. It boosts the ability of the liver and kidneys to filter toxins from the blood.

Milk thistle can be used to treat serious liver disorders like cirrhosis and hepatitis and, when taken regularly as part of a healthy diet and lifestyle, can return liver function to normal after several months. Milk thistle's remarkable detox properties are recommended for all heavy users of alcohol and pharmaceutical drugs that are hard on the liver, including chemotherapy

Milk thistle is best taken in capsule form with a daily dose of 100–200mg standardised for 70–80 percent silymarin. Available from health food stores and mail order suppliers. Milk thistle should not be taken in pregnancy.

Molybdenum

A trace mineral stored in the liver, bones and

kidneys and used in tiny amounts to metabolise iron and nitrogen. Molybdenum is essential to a healthy reproductive system and helps prevent sexual impotence in older men. The mineral is depleted by food refining and poor soil, so a diet high in refined and processed foods may cause a deficiency. Conversely, too high an intake of the mineral may cause an excess of uric acid in the body resulting in the painful condition of gout.

We need only a tiny amount of molybdenum daily and this should be obtainable from a reasonable diet. The mineral is included in some multimineral preparations at levels of around 100µg.

● *No official RDA in Britain, but in the USA the recommended levels are between 30–300µg for children depending on age, and 150–500µg for adults.*
Best food sources: Beans, cereal grains, peas, legumes and dark green leafy vegetables.

Multivitamins

A balanced diet with plenty of fresh fruit and vegetables should contain all the vitamins and minerals we need to keep healthy. However, there are times in life when we may need more nutrients than our diet provides, such as during or after illness, or when we are particularly stressed.

A multivitamin and mineral supplement is an easy and convenient way to guard against deficiencies and ensures a balanced intake of these important nutrients

Many groups of people require extra vitamins and minerals. These include anyone on a restricted diet (diabetics, vegans, food allergy sufferers), the elderly, people with poor appetites, convalescents, pregnant and breastfeeding women, smokers and drinkers (who need extra antioxidants), faddy eaters, slimmers, athletes and highly active people.

When choosing a multivitamin and mineral preparation, check that the product provides high levels of the main antioxidant nutrients – vitamins A, C, and E (with natural rather than synthetic vitamin E) and beta carotene, and that it gives 100 percent, or preferably more, of the recommended daily allowance (RDA) of other vitamins and minerals.

Mushrooms (Maitake, Reishi and Shiitake)

The **maitake** mushroom has a long history of use in China and Japan, and is both edible and medicinal. It is considered to be an adaptogen, helping the body cope with stress and normalising body functions. Research carried out in Japan suggests that maitake has strong anti-viral and anti-cancer properties and is a powerful immune stimulant. Maitake mushrooms can be bought fresh, dried, or in capsule, extract or tea form.

Reishi is a bitter-tasting Japanese mushroom that grows on trees in strange, woody formations. Non-toxic and cultivated solely for medicinal purposes, reishi is considered to be one of the most important tonics in Chinese medicine and to improve longevity. This unique mushroom's many health attributes include strengthening the immune system, protecting the liver, reducing inflammation and inhibiting the growth of some cancers.

Reishi is available in tablet or extract form from health food stores.

Shiitake is another Japanese mushroom which has been valued as a food and medicine for over 2000 years. Shiitake mushrooms contain vitamins, minerals, amino acids and special chemicals called polysaccharides, which are known to strengthen the immune system by increasing T-cell function. When sun-dried, shiitake mushrooms are a rich source of vitamin D. Shiitake extracts increase energy levels and resistance to disease, and lower blood pressure and cholesterol levels.

Shiitake mushrooms are available fresh or dried; extracts are sold in tablet or capsule form.

Niacin
(see Vitamin B3)

Vitamin P
(see Bioflavonoids)

PABA

Para-aminobenzoic acid (PABA) is an antioxidant nutrient and part of the structure of vitamin B9 (folic acid). It aids the assimilation of vitamin B5 (pantothenic acid) and may enhance the effect of hormones in the body. The nutrient has been used to treat and prevent abnormal fibrous tissue growths in some auto-immune and connective tissue disorders.

PABA is sometimes used as an ingredient in sunscreen lotions. High oral doses may be recommended for the skin condition vitiligo, in which patches of skin lose their pigmentation. PABA is known as the anti-grey hair vitamin, as some reports suggest it darkens grey hair if the loss of colour is caused by stress or a nutritional deficiency.

PABA is available in capsule form for specific needs. Small amounts of PABA are present in some B complex vitamin or multivitamin products.

● *No official RDA.* Best food sources: Liver, kidney, molasses, spinach, mushrooms and wholegrain cereals.

Pantothenic Acid
(see Vitamin B5)

Pau d'Arco

A South American herb also known as *lapacho*, with useful anti-fungal properties. A natural antibiotic and powerful antioxidant, natural health practitioners use pau d'arco internally and externally to treat local yeast infections and candidiasis. As a blood cleanser, the herb also helps to clear up various types of infection.

Pau d'arco is available from health food stores and herbalists. The recommended daily dose is between 500–3000mg.

Peppermint

Over the years, the peppermint herb has been used to treat various minor ailments including headaches, sore gums, circulatory and digestive disorders. Recent Danish research has shown that the oil distilled from the leaves of the plant is an effective natural remedy for irritable bowel syndrome. The oil's warming and soothing properties relax the smooth muscles in the gastro-intestinal tract and reduce the production of gas.

Peppermint can be taken as a fresh herb, dried in a tea, as a tincture, and as tablets and capsules of peppermint oil. The most effective therapeutic dose is about 200mg daily, taken as three or four capsules of peppermint oil, three times a day after meals.

Phosphatidylserine (PS)

An exciting new supplement that has been shown to restore memory in middle and old age, relieve depression and reduce stress-hormone production in athletes. Phosphatidylserine (PS) is a phosphorus-containing fat, found in all body cells. PS occurs in especially high concentrations in the brain, where it regulates mineral transfer and the transmission of electrical and chemical messages from one nerve cell to the next. It keeps the cell membranes flexible, ensuring easy passage of nutrients between the brain cells.

PS is made in the body from nutrients in our diet, notably methionine (an amino acid found in nuts, corn, rice, seeds, grains), vitamin B12 (eggs, fish, meat, dairy foods), essential fatty acids (oily fish, flax seed oil) and folic acid (leafy green vegetables).

Levels of PS decline with age (or nutrient deficiencies), causing the cell membranes to harden and lose their flexibility. This results in gradual loss of memory and concentration.

The new supplement is made by extracting PS from soya lecithin – an expensive and highly complex process. The supplement claims to increase the flexibility of hardened brain cell membranes, allowing nutrients to enter the cell more easily.

The dose for a middle-aged person wanting to prevent age-related brain degeneration, is one 100mg capsule each morning. To treat age-related memory impairment, one 100mg capsule should be taken two or three times daily for the first four to six weeks, reducing to a maintenance dose of 100mg daily. Available from selected health food stores and mail order suppliers.

Phosphorus

The mineral phosphorus is present in every cell in the body, and is involved in most of the body's physiological chemical reactions. Phosphorus is needed to form strong bones and teeth and to activate the B complex vitamins. To function efficiently, phosphorus needs calcium and vitamin D. Calcium and phosphorus should be balanced two to one to work correctly (twice as much calcium as phosphorus).

The mineral is not usually taken as a supplement on its own but as an ingredient in multivitamin and mineral preparations.

● *RDA is 800mg.*
Best food sources: Milk, canned fish and nuts.

Pollen
(see also Propolis/ Royal Jelly)

Granules or tablets prepared from the pollen collected by bees may help hayfever sufferers. As allergic reactions occasionally occur, it is important to read the manufacturer's advice for the product before using.

Potassium

Potassium is one of the most important minerals in the body. Its function is to control the fluid and acid/alkaline balance. It works with other minerals to form essential electrically charged ions known as 'electrolytes', that make up the fluids in the body. The balance of these electrolytes plays a vital role in cardiovascular health.

Potassium is crucial for many body functions, including nerve conduction, energy production, heartbeat, synthesis of nucleic acids and proteins, blood pressure, and muscle contraction.

If the body becomes dehydrated (due to chronic diarrhoea, vomiting, fasting, sweating, or diuretics), potassium levels may become seriously depleted, changing the body's chemistry and the electrolyte balance. Potassium is also lost through drinking large amounts of caffeinated drinks like cola and coffee and eating sugary foods. A deficiency of the mineral causes overwhelming fatigue, lowered blood pressure, muscle pains and vomiting.

The mineral is not usually taken as a supplement on its own, but may be prescribed to restore the body's electrolyte balance. Potassium is included in high potency multivitamin and mineral preparations.

● *No official RDA, but a daily intake of about 900mg from the diet is considered healthy.*

Best food sources:
Citrus fruits, watercress, and green leafy vegetables, bananas, potatoes, mint leaves and sunflower seeds.

Propolis
(see Pollen/Royal Jelly)

Propolis is the sticky 'glue' collected from plants and trees by bees which they use to build the beehive. Its amazing antibiotic and healing properties have been recognised since Roman times and are still not fully understood.

Propolis contains a wide variety of organic and amino acids, vitamins, minerals and most importantly bioflavonoids, believed to be the active ingredient in the healing process.

Traditionally used for healing sores and wounds and taken internally for coughs and sore throats, propolis also combats *Helicobacter pylori*, the bacteria causing peptic and duodenal ulcers.

Propolis is available in capsules or as a tincture to treat sore gums and mouth ulcers.

Psyllium Seed

A grain grown in India which is popularly used for its fibre content. Psyllium seed makes a good intestinal cleanser and stool softener. It promotes regular intestinal function and bowel movements, alleviating not only constipation, but also diarrhoea and haemorrhoids. Psyllium creates a feeling of fullness in the stomach, so is helpful to slimmers.

The grain is sold as dried seeds, wafers, powders and liquids. An average dose is one teaspoonful of powdered psyllium mixed with at least 285ml/8fl ozs of water or liquid, to be taken at mealtimes. The mixture thickens rapidly and should be taken immediately. It is important to drink plenty of water with psyllium to prevent it causing a blockage. Not to be taken during pregnancy.

Pycnogenol

Pycnogenol belongs to a group of substances called anthocyanidins, and is made from the nutrient-rich bark of maritime pine trees. Like other anthocyanidins, it is the subject of much ongoing research into its many health benefits, in particular, its role in the support of the capillaries (the tiny blood vessels) and the collagen from which they are formed.

Pycnogenol is a complex of about 40 natural ingredients and a rich source of vitamins, bioflavonoids, and more complex flavonoids, with anti-inflammatory and anti-viral properties

Pycnogenol is also a powerful antioxidant – its active ingredient is proanthocyanidin. Capsules are available from health food stores.

Pycnogenol should not be taken during pregnancy.

Pyridoxine
(see Vitamin B6)

Q10
(see Coenzyme Q10)

Quercetin

One of the bioflavonoids (special nutrients found with vitamin C in fruit and vegetables) that has antioxidant, anti-inflammatory and antihistamine properties. Quercetin may be helpful in preventing nerve, eye and kidney damage in those with diabetes.

Usually taken as part of a vitamin C supplement, along with other bioflavonoids like rutin.

Best food sources:
Onions, apples, tea, beans and leafy green vegetables.

Riboflavin
(see vitamin B2)

Royal Jelly
A bee product used as an energy-boosting tonic.

Prepared from the highly nutritious, milky salivary secretions of worker bees for the select bee larvae destined to develop into queen bees. The sterile worker bees never benefit from the substance they create, and live only about six weeks. By contrast, the queen bees which consume the jelly grow to twice the size of the worker bees and live for six years, laying up to 2000 eggs every day of their lives. No wonder royal jelly is hailed as a special tonic!

When taken daily for three to five months, royal jelly is claimed to rejuvenate the body and increase energy levels.

Analysis of royal jelly shows it contains only trace amounts of vitamins, minerals and various essential amino acids. However, research suggests that it is the balance of these nutrients that accounts for its supposedly beneficial effects. Royal jelly also contains *trans-l-hydroxydelta 2-decenoic acid*, a unique substance thought to account for the queen bee's longer lifespan

Royal jelly is available as fresh jelly capsules or freeze-dried (150g of royal jelly must be taken to have a beneficial effect). Royal jelly is also added to some supplement combinations.

Rutin

Rutin is one of the stronger bioflavonoids (nutrients found in fruit and vegetables that work synergistically with vitamin C) and is obtained from buckwheat and other sources. Like other bioflavonoids, it protects and strengthens the tiny blood vessels, so is a good choice of supplement for anyone with a tendency to bruise or bleed easily.

Rutin is also a successful treatment for bleeding gums and may ease the symptoms of hayfever and some inflammatory conditions.

Rutin is available as a supplement on its own or combined with other bioflavonoids and vitamin C. An effective daily dose is about 120mg.

St John's Wort
(also known as Hypericum)

A herb used in Europe as a topical wound healer for hundreds of years. St John's Wort is now enjoying renewed popularity as the 'sunshine' supplement because of its depression-lifting properties.

The herb's active ingredients include a substance called hypericin, which appears to regulate levels of certain brain chemicals, in the same way that allopathic medications like Prozac do. The antidepressant effects may not be felt until the herb has been taken daily for about a month. A small number of people may initially experience mild nausea, tiredness or lack of appetite, but these symptoms soon disappear.

The recommended dose is two tablets daily of a standardised extract containing 0.3 percent hypericin. Higher doses may result in a photosensitivity reaction in some people.

St John's Wort is available from health food stores and from mail order suppliers. It should not be taken with tyramine-containing foods, such as mature cheeses, red meats and wines, nor by pregnant or breastfeeding women.

Saw Palmetto

A herb favoured by the North American Indians and taken as part of their diet. Herbalists and naturopaths in Europe and America have long used saw palmetto berries to treat problems of the genito-urinary tract in both men and women. Saw palmetto acts as a urinary antiseptic and diuretic,

so is an effective remedy for conditions such as 'honeymoon cystitis'. In recent years, saw palmetto has become the leading herbal remedy for preventing and relieving symptoms caused by an enlarged prostate gland – a common problem in middle-aged and older men. It helps reduce the frequency of night-time urination and improves urine flow. The herb may also stimulate the appetite and improve sexual function and libido.

Saw palmetto is sold in capsule form at most health food stores.

Selenium
(see also Trace Minerals)

An important antioxidant trace mineral that works in conjunction with vitamin E. Selenium boosts the immune system, keeps the liver healthy and helps to combat the ageing process. Selenium is also needed to make thyroxine, the thyroid gland hormone regulating metabolism.

Selenium occurs naturally in the soil and enters the food chain through plants. Populations of countries with naturally low levels of selenium, or where intensive farming methods have depleted the mineral in the soil, may be linked to an increased risk of cancer and heart disease. The selenium content of the average daily diet varies enormously: over 350µg in Venezuela; more than 200µg in parts of the USA, Thailand and Japan; 175µg in Greece and only 31µg in Great Britain.

Many multivitamin preparations include selenium. These are intended to make good any deficiency in the diet rather than to have a therapeutic effect. Larger amounts of selenium (up to 200µg daily) have been found to benefit arthritis sufferers because the mineral helps the body to make anti-inflammatory substances called prostaglandins.

Selenium supplements are available in tablet form and are often combined with other antioxidant vitamins like vitamin E.

● *RDA is between 60 and 200µg.*

Best food sources: Meat (especially kidney and liver), fish, shellfish, yeast, eggs, garlic, dairy products and wholemeal bread and grains.

Shark Cartilage

The tough skeleton of the shark is dried and pulverised to a fine powder to make this unusual supplement, which may be of value in a number of serious disorders. Shark cartilage contains an angiogenesis inhibitor (a component that suppresses the development of new blood vessels). This may shrink some types of cancerous growths by depriving them of their blood supply. Certain eye diseases such as macular degeneration and diabetic retinopathy are characterised by new blood vessels growing in inappropriate areas within the eye. These may also respond to supplements of shark cartilage.

Other conditions helped by this unusual remedy include inflammation of the lining of the bowel, psoriasis and arthritis.

Shark cartilage is available in powder and capsule form from some health food stores and by mail order. Check that the product contains 100 percent shark cartilage, as quality processing and purity are essential to its effectiveness. This supplement should not be taken by children or pregnant women, by athletes in training or by anyone who has suffered a heart attack. or had recent surgery. It would be wise to consult a nutritionally-orientated doctor for advice before taking shark cartilage.

Shark Liver Oil

An old established health product used for years in Norway and Sweden as a general tonic and to promote healing of wounds and irritations of the respiratory tract. Modern research shows that shark liver oil contains two important constituents: alkylglycerols and squalene.

Alkylglycerols occur in small amounts in mother's milk, bone marrow, the liver and spleen. They are involved in producing white blood cells and play an important role in the functioning of the immune system.

Squalene, is an unsaturated fatty material, widely distributed in nature and occurring in large concentrations in shark liver oil. It is a well-known ingredient in beauty creams and ointments and an effective ulcer-healing treatment. Squalene exerts a positive effect on the liver and immune system and protects the skin from ultra-violet exposure. When taken orally, it is quickly absorbed and transformed into bile acids in the liver and targeted to fatty tissues in the body.

Capsules are available from health food stores and by mail order.

Siberian Ginseng

Siberian Ginseng is prepared from the roots of the *Eleutherococcus senticocus* plant, and is related to the Panax American or Korean ginsengs but is from a different botanical family.

Siberian ginseng's main use is as a tonic, strengthening and normalising all the body systems. The herb's antioxidants and other compounds boost the immune system and increase energy and endurance levels. Health problems such as lack of energy, stress, bronchitis, circulatory problems and infertility may be improved by Siberian ginseng. Not only does the herb strengthen the adrenal and reproductive glands, but it also helps the body adapt to difficult or demanding situations.

Many herbalists consider Siberian ginseng to be the most suitable type of ginseng for women, as its natural plant oestrogens are helpful in controlling menopausal problems like hot flushes.

The herb is best taken first thing in the morning, as its effect on sleep is similar to caffeine. It is not recommended for anyone with high blood pressure or an irregular heartbeat, nor should it be taken by pregnant women or nursing mothers.

Siberian ginseng is available from health food stores, pharmacies and mail order suppliers in various forms, including capsules, tablets, whole root, slices, liquid and herbal combinations.

Silicon

Silicon (also known as silica) is the most plentiful element on the planet after oxygen. Chemical fertilisers and food refining tend to deplete it in food crops.

In the body, silicon is a vital part of connective tissues, bones, blood vessels and cartilage. It helps strengthen the condition of the skin, hair and nails by improving production of collagen and keratin, the proteins found in the joints, hair and nails.

Silicon supplements are usually prepared from horsetail or bamboo plants and some preparations are available in gel form. These protect the lining of the stomach and intestines and are an effective treatment for gastritis, irritable bowel syndrome, flatulence and heartburn. The gel can also be applied to the gums to treat gingivitis and mouth ulcers, or used on the skin for chronic skin conditions like psoriasis and acne.

Best food sources: Root vegetables and other forms of plant fibre, vegetables and fruit grown organically, brown rice and hard drinking water.

Slippery Elm

A traditional remedy made from the inner bark of the tree and used to soothe inflamed mucous membranes in the stomach, bowels and urinary tract. Its soothing properties also help diarrhoea, stomach ulcers, colds, 'flu and sore throats.

The powdered bark can be added to liquid to make a healing drink.

Slow-release vitamins

Some supplements are labelled 'slow release' or 'sustained release', and claim to release their ingredients into the body over a period hours. As absorption of any nutrient depends on how well it is digested as well as the dose, the efficacy claims of some of these products may be questionable.

Supplements of water-soluble vitamins B and C are most likely to offered in this format. Products are presented as capsules containing tiny 'beads' of nutrients, or as specially coated tablets which slowly erode as they pass through through the digestive processes.

Sodium

The adult body contains approximately 100g of sodium, half of which is located in the cells of the bones and tissue fluids. Working with potassium, sodium regulates the body's electrolyte and acid-alkali balances, the conduction of the nerves, muscle contractions, and the production of amino acids and adrenaline.

About 3g of sodium is required daily to carry out these functions, but most people consume considerably more than this. Salt (in the form of sodium chloride), is added to a huge number of foods, making it difficult to have a controlled intake.

It has been estimated that about half our salt intake comes from processed foods and soft drinks and half from salt added when preparing and serving food at home. Only a small amount of the day's consumption comes from the natural sodium content of foods.

Too much salt depletes potassium levels in the body and increases the risk of high blood pressure in people predisposed to hypertension. While most excess sodium is excreted via the urine, high intakes can lead to a build-up of fluid in the body and be a contributory factor in migraine. It is a wise parent who discourages a liking for salty foods in their children from an early age, and so limits overall intake.

Best food sources: Sea salt, shellfish, carrots, artichokes, offal and bacon.

Spirulina

Spirulina (like chlorella) is one of the new green 'superfoods' derived from fresh water algae and available in tablet or powdered food form. Spirulina contains significant amounts of a wide range of nutrients and enzymes including chlorophyll, vitamins, iron and selenium and is a good source of plant protein and the fatty acid GLA. To obtain maximum nutritional benefit, 20g of spirulina should be taken daily. Powdered spirulina is more economical than tablets.

A potent new form, *Hawaiian Pacifica Spirulina* claims to be the first totally organic spirulina. It contains two to five times more vitamin B12 than a portion of liver, so makes an ideal supplement for vegans and vegetarians who may be deficient in this nutrient.

The same product also claims to help with weight control, as it suppresses the appetite when taken 30 minutes before a meal.

Various brands of spirulina are available from health food stores and pharmacies.

Starflower Oil
(see also Borage)

Starflower oil provides a richer source of gamma linolenic acid (GLA) than is found in evening primrose oil. GLA is an unusual fatty acid with no normal dietary source (the body makes it from linoleic acid found in vegetable oils). GLA has a regulatory effect on the immune system, the circulation and the menstrual cycle. The benefits of starflower oil have not been fully researched, although the oil's chemical structure is quite different from that of evening primrose oil, another valuable source of GLA.

Borage (starflower oil) supplements may be taken singly or combined with evening primrose oil or other nutrients.

Sulphur

A trace element required by the body in minute amounts to create healthy skin and hair. Found naturally in the diet in all high protein foods and in nutrients such as amino acids and the B complex vitamins, thiamin and biotin. Sulphur is not available as a food supplement but may be found in topical skin creams and ointments.

Best food sources: Lean beef, fish, eggs and cabbage.

Superoxide Dismutase *(SOD)*

An antioxidant enzyme which becomes increasingly active as a defence mechanism when free radical levels are raised in the body. The SOD enzyme is one of the most commonly occurring body proteins after collagen, albumin, globulin and haemoglobin. Levels of SOD tend to decline as we get older, while free radical production increases. SOD is particularly important because it neutralises the most common free radical, superoxide, which may also be the most dangerous.

SOD occurs in two forms, one requiring copper and zinc to function, and the other manganese.

SOD is available as a supplement from health food stores.

Best food sources: Most green plants including barley grass, wheat grass, broccoli, Brussels sprouts, and cabbage.

Thiamin
(see Vitamin B1)

Trace Minerals

The name for the vital mineral nutrients required by the body in minute amounts for the maintenance of health. These include chromium, copper, iodine, iron, manganese, molybdenum, selenium, silicon, sulphur and zinc.

By contrast, the body requires substantial amounts of the major minerals calcium, magnesium, phosphorus and potassium.

Tryptophan

Tryptophan is one of eight essential amino acids (proteins found in food that cannot be manufactured by the body). It is used as a natural sleeping aid as it has tranquillising properties. A few years ago, some tryptophan supplements became contaminated in manufacture. This caused a health scare and the supplement was taken off the shelves. Now Solgar have launched a new safe form of tryptophan called 5-hydroxytryptophan (5-HTP). derived from *Griffonia simplicifolia*, a small African bean

Best food sources:
Peanuts and peanut butter, foods low in fat and protein but high in carbohydrate.

Ubiquinone
(see Coenzyme Q10)

Uva Ursi

Also known as *bearberry*, The herb has diuretic properties and has been used by both sexes to treat urinary and kidney infections. Men find it helps alleviate prostate disorders. Uva ursi may also be helpful for treating disorders of the liver, pancreas, spleen and small intestine.

Uva ursi is available in capsule form from health food stores and herbalists and should be taken up to three times a day to relieve symptoms.

Vanadium

A little-known trace mineral, believed to inhibit the formation of cholesterol in the blood vessels. It may also help reduce high blood sugar and prevent tooth decay. High doses are toxic and may cause manic depression. Vanadium is included in some of the newer multi-vitamin and mineral preparations.

Best food sources: Parsley, seafood and fish.

Valerian

A popular natural remedy for anyone suffering from anxiety-related insomnia. This popular herb has various other useful applications. It soothes nervousness and irritable bowel syndrome, eases menstrual pain, muscle cramps and spasms.

Valerian is available as a tea or in capsules from health food stores and pharmacies.

Wheat Grass

An excellent source of B complex and other vitamins, minerals and trace elements. It is said that one pound of wheat grass is the nutritional equivalent of 25 pounds of the best quality fruit and vegetables. Wheat grass is one of the best-known sources of chlorophyll, a plant pigment which contains minerals, and is highly cleansing and alkalising, helping to build up resistance to infection. Sprouted wheat grass can be juiced or obtained in powder or tablet form from health food stores

White Willow

The bark of the white willow tree *(Salix alba)* has been used for thousands of years to alleviate pain and fever. It contains salicin, which is similar to aspirin in action, although weaker. Unlike aspirin, white willow benefits from tannins, which are helpful to digestion. The herb's analgesic actions are slower-acting but last longer than standard aspirin products, providing a gentle remedy for pain and inflammation generally. White willow's main components (salicin, quercetin and tannins) help relieve headaches, backache and toothache.

The herb is available from health food stores

and herbalists in the form of a tea, tincture or tablet, standardised for salicin content. Long term use may cause gastrointestinal irritation. White willow should not be taken by children or anyone allergic to aspirin.

Notes about aspirin:
Aspirin, one of the world's most widely-used medicines, is a synthetic derivative of white willow bark. Chemists made a small change to the bark's active component to create acetylsalicylic acid, better known as aspirin.

Research suggests that, in addition to relieving fever, inflammation and pain, the humble aspirin has other remarkable health benefits. Taking half a tablet a day with food (to spare stomach irritation) decreases the stickiness of the blood and the risk of heart attacks and strokes. A small regular dose of aspirin reduces the risk of cancer of the colon, lung and oesophagus and may protect against Alzheimer's disease.

Anyone considering a low dose aspirin regime should discuss it with their doctor first. Aspirin does not suit everyone and should not be taken by children, nursing mothers or those on blood-thinning drugs.

Wild Yam

Wild yam remedies are derived from the plant's long, twisting roots (rhizomes) and have long been used in Asia as a liver tonic, digestive aid and muscle relaxant.

Animal studies have shown that the steroidal saponins found in wild yam may ease the pain and stiffness associated with rheumatoid arthritis. Extracts of the plant have been found to relieve headaches,

joint and muscle pains. Wild yam contains diosgenin, a steroid precursor, which is used in the laboratory to make 'natural progesterone' and other hormonal products – to relieve adverse symptoms of PMS and the menopause.

Ordinary yam creams and other over the counter products *do not* contain or convert into progesterone or dehydroepiandrosterone (DHEA) in the body, but provide a useful form of plant oestrogens.

Wild yam extract is available in health stores as a cream, tincture, tablet or capsule.

Special notes about wild yam and natural progesterone:

Unique skin creams containing pharmaceutical grade progesterone or combined hormones, are prepared from wild yam extract or the soya plant. Known as *natural progesterone,* they are used by many women as an alternative to orthodox hormone replacement therapy and to treat other health symptoms. (The medical journal *The Lancet*, reported that wild yam may help reverse the effects of osteoporosis.)

In the UK, natural progesterone cream is available only from selected outlets or by private prescription (see page 91).

Zinc

Zinc is a trace mineral, essential to over 80 body processes and helps maintain a healthy immune system. The body uses the mineral for tissue repair and renewal, so a zinc supplement will promote healing and may even improve the the condition of the skin in cases of acne.

Human fertility is also affected by zinc levels in the body: Low levels in

men may result in reduced sperm count; while pregnant women deficient in zinc are more likely to give birth to smaller babies. Zinc deficiency also causes loss of taste and smell, and may well be a contributory factor in *anorexia nervosa,* the slimmer's disease. A poor appetite is often one of the first signs of a zinc deficiency.

To top up dietary levels, 5 to 10mg of organic or chelated zinc should be taken daily. Zinc is usually included in multimineral supplements. Other useful zinc products include zinc lozenges, an effective remedy for sore throats, and zinc and castor oil cream to prevent and treat nappy rash.

● *RDA 15mg.*

Best food sources:
Oysters, sardines and other seafoods, baker's yeast, wholemeal bread, nuts, seeds, beef, liver, eggs and cheese.

Useful addresses

The following companies provide a wide range of general and specialist health products on request. Brochures are available on request.

Bionaire
Lakeside, 180 Lifford
Lane, Kings Norton,
Birmingham B30 3NT
Tel 0121 451 5572
Fax 0121 451 3879

Nature's Best
1 Lamberate...
Tunbridge...
Kent TN4 ...
Tel 0892 ...
Fax 0892 ...

Larkhall Green Farm
Natural Health Products
225 Putney Bridge Road
London SW15 2PY
Tel 081-874 1130
Fax 081-871 9690

**Life and Soul Pouch
Nutrition**
(Women's supplements)
30 St Gabriels Manor,
Cormont Road,

**More information
and a wide range of nutritional products available from:**

GRAMPIAN HEALTH FOODS
5 Crown Street
Aberdeen
Aberdeenshire
AB11 6HA
Tel: 01224 590886
www.grampianhealthfoods.co.uk

Grampian Health Foods is the exclusive stockist in Aberdeen of the **viridian** range of nutritional supplements. Founded in 1999, **viridian** has been named the leading brand of ethical vitamins, by *Here's Health* magazine, due to the company's commitment to green business practice, purity of ingredients, recycling scheme and charity donation programme.

London SE5 9RH
Tel/fax 0171-582 2871